Leptin Diet:

21 Leptin Resistance Recipes For Rapid Weight Loss

Table of content

Introduction

Leptin is a hormone which triggers a feeling of fullness and prompts the body to stop eating. It is thought that, for many obese people, their sensitivity to leptin has become reduced, meaning that they continue to eat even when they have consumed enough calories. This causes a vicious circle in which, as their weight continues to increase, it takes more and more food to make them feel satisfied. Being obese suppresses leptin function, meaning that obese people genuinely feel more hunger than non-obese people — it is not simply a case of greed or willpower. It is very hard to override these feelings of hunger, which is why so many diets fail — it is estimated by some sources that in 90% of cases, dieters regain the lost weight within a few years. This is because a constant state of hunger and dissatisfaction is impossible to live with for the rest of your life.

The leptin diet is designed to reset this imbalance, meaning that a healthy amount of calories is all that is required to make you feel full and satisfied. As your body fat decreases, your leptin function should improve and so make it possible to maintain your weight loss for the rest of your life.

The leptin diet has a few basic rules to help you lose weight effectively:

Rule One: Eat three meals a day, with no snacking in between. It is very easy to allow extra food to creep in to your diet, and this will interrupt the natural cycle of eating out of hunger. If you eat out of boredom or as a "treat" you will stop your leptin levels from balancing, and you may experience cravings and side effects such as lethargy and headaches. Plan and eat three healthy meals, and you will find yourself becoming satisfied with the food you consume and not seeking to 'top up' in between.

Rule Two: Eat your final meal at least three hours before you go to bed. This will give your food time to digest before your metabolism experiences its natural dip while you sleep, and reduce the amount of calories that are laid down as fat. Many people find that they eat their main meal of the day at night time — if at all possible, try to change this so that you are either eating three even-sized meals, or your main meal becomes your breakfast or lunch.

Rule Three: Control your portion sizes. A large meal will overload your system and mean that you require greater volumes the next time you eat in order to trigger your feeling of fullness. Retrain your body to be happy with smaller amounts of food. Eat slowly, so that your stomach has time to register the food you have consumed — this usually takes around twenty minutes, so give yourself enough time to genuinely feel full. Unfortunately, many people have been 'programmed' since childhood to consume all of the food on their plate and to override any feelings of fullness that your body is naturally sending your brain.

Rule Four: Make sure you consume protein for breakfast. Many traditional breakfast foods such as cereal or toast concentrate on carbohydrates which are quickly digested and will rapidly leave you feeling hungry again. Eggs are a perfect breakfast food and will help stave off hunger until your next meal time. You can also consume meat such as chicken or beef for breakfast, or

Rule Five: Reduce carbohydrates in your diet. Our bodies are designed to crave carbohydrates, since they are an easy way to pack in calories and lay down fat, which is a natural advantage if food is scarce. However, in our current food-rich environment, it is not useful and rapidly leads to obesity. You should reduce your intake of carbohydrates to high fiber foods such as fruit, vegetables and whole grains. It is not necessary to eliminate carbs entirely, since this can make it hard to consume sufficient vitamins and fiber, but avoid refined foods such as white bread, pasta and sugar.

Also, try to avoid diet sodas and commercially packaged "diet foods". These can trick your body into thinking it is consuming sugar, and will trigger a craving response when the effect wears off. Although they will not cause weight gain in themselves, they will make it harder to stick to your new healthy food patterns.

Exercise is a vital part of a healthy lifestyle. It is safe to continue an existing exercise regime, or undertake a light exercise programme, but the first few weeks of a new diet are probably not the time to start a new high-intensity fitness programme. Save this until your new diet plan becomes established and you feel happy with the amount you are consuming.

If you stick to the leptin diet, you should begin to notice positive effects such as weight loss, better sleep and increased energy. You will find that you feel full after smaller amounts of food and you will find cravings for sugar and carbohydrate heavy foods are reduced.

Chapter 1 – Prawn and Coconut Rice

<u>You will need:</u>

2 tablespoons of olive oil

1 white onion, diced

2 red or yellow peppers, diced

6 cloves of garlic, minced

1 teaspoon of fresh ginger, minced

2 large tomatoes, peeled and diced

1/4 cup of unsweetened, grated coconut

1 3/4 cups of basmati rice

3 cups of water

1 cup of low fat Vanilla Yogurt

1/2 cup of chopped parsley

Salt and pepper to taste

16-20 large prawns, peeled and deveined

Bamboo skewers

<u>Method:</u>

Soak 6 wooden skewers in water for 20-30 minutes to prevent them from burning.

Heat the olive oil in a large sauté pan (fitted with a lid) over medium-high heat. Add the onion and peppers and cook for 5 minutes, until onion is translucent. Stir in the garlic and ginger and cook until fragrant. Add the tomatoes and coconut and mix well. Cook for another 5 minutes.

Add the rice and stir frequently until lightly browned, about 2 minutes. Add the water and stir well to combine. Bring to a boil and reduce heat to low. Cover and let it simmer for 15-20 minutes.

Remove from the heat. In a small bowl, temper the yogurt (to prevent splitting) by adding some of the rice mixture to the yogurt and stirring. Continue adding rice mixture gradually and stirring until yogurt is warmed through. Mix the entire bowl of yogurt into the rice mixture. Add the parsley and salt and pepper to taste and fold together to combine. Thread about 4 shrimp per skewer, through both the head and tail. Grill over medium heat for 1-2 minutes per side. Shrimp should be thoroughly cooked through and firm and white in the center.

Chapter 2 – Kale Salad

<u>You will need:</u>

1 Bunch of Organic Kale, roughly chopped

Half a tin of Organic Cooked Chickpeas, drained

1/3 of Small Sweet Onion (Thinly Sliced)

1/3 Cup of Raisins

<u>For the dressing:</u>

A tablesoon of Organic Sesame Tahini

The juice of one lemon

A pinch Of Cayenne or Paprika (adjust the heat to your personal taste)

1 teaspoon of Salt

<u>Method:</u>

Combine the first four ingredients, then combine the dressing ingredients and pour over. Serve immediately. If you want to make this salad as a packed lunch, store the dressing in a small, watertight jar and dress the salad just before you eat it.

Chapter 3 – Tomato Borscht

<u>You will need:</u>

2 Tablespoons of Olive Oil

1 Small Sized Onion (Chopped)

1 Clove of Garlic (Chopped)

225g of Raw Beetroot (Peeled & Grated)

1 Teaspoon of Ground Toasted Cumin Seeds

1/4 Teaspoon of Ground Cinnamon

225g of Ripe Fresh Tomatoes (Chopped)

250 ml of Tomato Juice

1 Tablespoon Of Sun-Dried Tomatoes (Chopped — this is optional)

600 ml of Vegetable Stock

1 Tablespoon Of Light Soy Sauce

Salt and pepper

<u>Method:</u>

Heat up a heavy pan and cook the olive oil, onions and garlic. Add the beetroot after 5 minutes. Wait until brown, then add everything else except for the soy sauce. Allow to cook this mixture for about 15 minutes before adding everything else. Add salt and pepper to taste — the soy sauce has a high level of salt, so you may not need to add any additional. Serve chilled or warm depending on your preference.

You can serve this soup scattered with cumin seeds and a swirl of soured cream.

Chapter 4 – Lentil and Quinoa Salad

<u>You will need:</u>

1 cup organic lentils, rinsed. Puy is best.

3 teaspoons of salt

1 cup of organic quinoa, rinsed

3 tablespoons of balsamic vinegar

3 tablespoons of organic extra virgin olive oil

1 whole organic plum tomato, diced

1 whole organic avocado, halved, pitted, peeled, diced

1 to 2 teaspoons of minced fresh coriander

2 tablespoons of lemon zest

Freshly ground pepper

<u>Method:</u>

Place lentils in a pot and add enough water to cover them by 2 inches. Stir in 1 teaspoon salt and bring to a boil. Reduce to a simmer and cook for 10 to 15 minutes, or until tender.

While lentils are cooking, cook quinoa with remaining salt according to package directions.

Drain lentils well and transfer to a bowl. Add quinoa and stir to combine. Let the mixture cool.

In a separate bowl, whisk together the vinegar and olive oil to make a vinaigrette. Add tomatoes and avocados to lentil mixture and drizzle with vinaigrette. Sprinkle with coriander, black pepper and lemon zest to serve.

Chapter 5 – Spicy Chicken Chili

<u>You will need:</u>

1 tablespoon of olive oil

 500g of skinless chicken breast, cubed

1 cup of onions, diced

400g of tinned tomatoes

400g tin of white beans

2 cloves of garlic, minced

1 fresh jalapeno, seeded and diced (if you prefer a spicier dish, leave the seeds in)

2 tablespoon of chili powder (adjust to taste)

1/2 teaspoon of dried oregano or a few sprigs of fresh

1/4 teaspoon of ground cumin

Salt and pepper to taste

<u>Method:</u>

Coat a large frying pan with olive oil. Add the chicken and onions and brown the chicken over low-medium heat until cooked through. Add all other ingredients and cook on low heat for approximately 15 to 20 minutes.

To increase spiciness, add red pepper flakes and/or diced green chilies to taste. You may also top with fresh coriander after cooking. Serve with brown rice or a crunchy green salad.

Chapter 6 – Salmon Fillets with Asparagus

<u>You will need:</u>

4 salmon fillets

1 tablespoon of chopped fresh rosemary or 1 teaspoon of dried

1 teaspoon of salt

500g — 750g of fresh asparagus spears

1 1/2 tablespoons of extra-virgin olive oil

1 small organic onion, diced

2 tablespoons of pine nuts

1 cup of water

1/2 cup of brown rice

<u>Method:</u>

Season the salmon with half the rosemary and 1/2 teaspoon salt. Allow to stand for 20 minutes and up to 1 hour before cooking. Preheat the oven to 425 degrees.

Add 1 cup of water to the pot and bring to a boil. Add 1/2 cup of brown rice, set to low and cover. Rice will be done in 35-40 minutes.

Snap the bottom of the asparagus ends to remove the woody ends. Season the asparagus with 1/2 teaspoon salt and some olive oil, toss to combine. Bake the asparagus for about 8-10 minutes at 425 degrees on a lined baking tray.

Heat 1 tablespoon of olive oil in a large wide saucepan over medium heat. Add the diced onion and cook, stirring occasionally, until translucent — this should take about 3 to 4 minutes. Add the pine nuts and the remaining rosemary. Cook, stirring continuously, until the pine nuts are fragrant and beginning to brown; around 3 to 5 minutes.

Remove the pine nuts and heat the remaining oil in the pan over medium-high heat. Add salmon, skinned-side up, and cook until golden brown, 3 to 5 minutes. Turn the salmon over, remove the pan from the heat and let stand until just cooked through, 3 to 5 minutes more.

Serve with a scoop of brown rice on bottom, topped with salmon and spoon the pine nuts and any liquid remaining in the pan over the salmon.

Chapter 7 – Filled Avocado

<u>You will need:</u>

1 ripe avocado

A tablespoon of 2% cottage cheese

Small tomato, diced

A lemon wedge

Sea salt and pepper

<u>Method:</u>

Carefully cut the avocado in half and scoop out the pit. Fill avocado halves with cottage cheese. Top with tomato, lemon juice, and sprinkle of salt.

Chapter 8 – Zingy Fish Tacos

<u>You will need:</u>

1 pound of 1-inch thick fish fillets — halibut, cod or other firm white fish will do

The juice of 2 limes

A bunch of chopped fresh coriander

1/4 cup of olive oil

1/4 cup of prepared salsa verde or pesto

1 jalepeno, diced (optional)

1/4 cup of mayonnaise (full fat)

1 teaspoon of sea salt, divided

1 cup of shredded green cabbage

1 cup of shredded red cabbage

2 small avocados, sliced

 8 whole wheat flour tortillas

2 limes, cut in half

<u>Method:</u>

Preheat grill to medium-high heat. Combine the lime juice, coriander, oil and fish fillets in large zip top bag; marinate in refrigerator for 20 minutes.

For a creamy salsa verde, combine salsa or pesto and mayonnaise in mini food processor or blender. Add jalepeno (optional). Puree until smooth.

Remove the fish from the marinade, season with 1/2 teaspoon sea salt, and place on hot grill pan. Grill fish for 6 minutes on each side and remove. Let it rest for several minutes then flake the fish with fork.

Place the lime halves on the grill pan, flesh side down, along with tortillas for 1 minute or until limes are grill marked and one side of tortillas are toasted. Remove and bend tortillas, toasted side out, into taco-shape.

Fill each tortilla with 1/4 cup of slaw and 2 slices of avocado. Divide the fish evenly among the tacos and drizzle each with 1 tablespoon sauce. Sprinkle with the remaining sea salt and serve with grilled lime half.

Chapter 9 – Goat's Cheese and Beetroot Winter Salad

<u>You will need:</u>

4 medium sized beetroots

2 cups fresh baby spinach

150g goat cheese (either hard or creamy — whichever you prefer)

1/2 small red onion, thinly sliced

1/2 cup of pine nuts (optional)

1 tablespoon of olive oil

<u>For the Dressing</u>

1 Tablespoon of extra virgin olive oil

2 Tablespoons of white balsamic vinegar (or lemon juice)

1 Teaspoon of dried oregano or a few sprigs of fresh oregano

Salt and pepper to taste

<u>Method:</u>

Preheat the oven to 375°. Place the beets in a shallow baking dish and pour over half the olive oil. Roll the beets to coat, and cover with a lid or aluminium foil. Bake until they are tender, which should take about an hour and thirty minutes. Remove from the oven and allow to cool. Once cool enough to handle, skin the beets, and cut into 1 inch pieces.

Mix the dressing ingredients together and set aside. Assemble the salad by dividing the greens between two salad plates. Arrange the beet slices and onion slices on top. Drizzle the dressing on top, just enough on each plate to lightly coat. Crumble the goat cheese, and garnish each plate with the goat cheese crumbles.

Chapter 10 – Beef Burritos

<u>You will need:</u>

1/2 cup of tomato salsa

1/2 cup of water

1/4 cup of uncooked long grain brown rice

400g can of black beans

300g of strip steak, trimmed and thinly sliced crosswise

1 tablespoon of olive oil

4 8-inch whole-wheat tortillas

1/2 cup of grated strong cheese, such as mature cheddar

1 avocado cut into slices

2 tablespoons of coarsely chopped fresh coriander

<u>For the Marinade:</u>

2 jalapenos, seeded and diced

A tablespoon of cumin seeds, toasted

Two tablespoons of olive oil

1 bunch of coriander (stems and leaves)

1 teaspoon of salt

1 tablespoon of cracked black pepper

1 clove of garlic, crushed

The juice of one lime

<u>Method:</u>

Put all the marinade ingredients in a blender, blend until smooth, and pour over beef slices. Cover and keep in refrigerator for at least one hour or overnight.

Cook the rice as per packet directions. When there is 10 minutes left of cooking time, add the salsa and water to rice and simmer for 5 minutes. Stir in the beans and simmer uncovered until the rice is tender and most of the liquid is absorbed, this should take about 5 minutes more.

Meanwhile, heat the oil in a large pan over medium-high heat. Add the steak slices and cook, stirring occasionally, until browned and cooked through to taste, 3 to 5 minutes.

To assemble, divide the steak among the tortillas and top with equal amounts of cheese, guacamole, chopped coriander and the rice mixture. Roll each tortilla into a burrito and eat straight away.

Chapter 11 – Turkey Burgers

<u>You will need:</u>

500g of ground turkey mince

1 cup of marinara sauce

1/4 cup of gouda cheese, grated

 1/4 cup of Mozzarella cheese, grated

Whole grain pita wraps

<u>To top burger:</u>

 salad greens (lettuce, cucumber, radishes, etc)

chopped red onion

Salt and pepper to taste

<u>Method:</u>

Mix all the ingredients with the ground turkey except the red onion and salad greens. Make into 4 individual patties and place on a lined baking sheet. Bake at 420 degrees for 15 minutes or grill until cooked through — check the centres to make sure the burgers are fully cooked.

Top with red onions and salad greens and serve in a pita or bun. You can adapt this recipe to make smaller turkey meatballs and serve in a tomato sauce.

Chapter 12 – Kale Crisps

These make an ideal crunchy treat to eat with fresh salsa or hummus.

<u>You will need:</u>

1 bunch of fresh kale

Cold-pressed, extra virgin olive oil

Sea salt

<u>Method:</u>

Preheat your oven to 350°F. Wash the kale in a tub full of water and then drain.

Cut or tear out the tough center stem, then tear the kale into 3-inch pieces. Dry the kale thoroughly, using a salad spinner, paper, or kitchen towels.

Place the kale in one layer on a baking sheet and drizzle a little extra virgin olive oil on each piece, massage it in, then lightly salt. Don't allow the kale to overlap or it will not become crisp.

Bake until the kale is crisp — it should take about 5 minutes. To stop it from burning, turn the baking sheet and check after 3 minutes. Remove the crisps from the oven and let them cool.

Chapter 13 – High Protein Morning Smoothie

<u>You will need:</u>

1 scoop whey protein powder

2 big handfuls fresh spinach

1 pear or ½ cup pineapple chunks

1 cup skimmed milk (you can substitute any milk; almond, rice, soy or coconut milk).

<u>Method:</u>

Add the ingredients to your blender in this order: milk, protein powder, spinach, fruit. Blend well and drink straight away.

Chapter 14 – Choc Chunk Cookies

<u>You will need:</u>

7 tablespoons palm shortening

1/3 cup plus 2 tablespoons of coconut sugar

1 tablespoon of raw honey

1 large egg

1/3 cup of coconut flour

1/3 cup of tapioca flour

1/3 cup of arrowroot flour

1/2 teaspoon of sea salt

1 teaspoon of baking soda

3/4 teaspoon of unflavoured gelatin powder

1 cup of carob chips or chunks

<u>Method:</u>

Preheat the oven to 350°F and adjust the rack to the middle position.

Place the palm shortening, sugar and honey in the bowl of a food processor. Beat on medium-high for 2 minutes. Scrape the sides of the bowl and mix in the egg. Sift the coconut flour, tapioca flour, arrowroot flour, sea salt, baking soda and gelatin into a large mixing bowl. With mixer on low, slowly add dry mixture to wet mixture. Stir in the carob chips.

Using a 1 1/2 tablespoon cookie scoop, scoop dough balls onto a baking sheet lined with parchment paper. Bake for 11 minutes.

If you want to store these cookies, place the uncooked scoops of dough onto a lined baking sheet and freeze until solid. Transfer the frozen balls to a sealed tub to store. When you want to cook them, space them out on a braking tray and cook from frozen for around 15 minutes.

Chapter 15 – Grilled Chicken Breasts with Tomato Salsa

<u>You will need:</u>

250g of cherries, pitted

1 small chopped white onion

1 large ripe tomato, cored and roughly chopped

3/4 teaspoon of salt, divided

1/2 teaspoon of ground black pepper, divided

2 tablespoons of chopped fresh coriander

2 tablespoons of whole wheat breadcrumbs

4 boneless, skinless chicken breasts. Pound between two sheets of clingfilm to flatten, using a heavy bottomed saucepan or rolling pin.

 2 tablespoons of extra-virgin olive oil

<u>Method</u>

Put the cherries, onion, tomato, 1/4 teaspoon salt and 1/4 teaspoon pepper into a food processor and pulse to make a chunky salsa. (Or, finely chop all of the ingredients and toss together in a bowl.) Stir in the coriander and set aside.

Put the breadcrumbs into a wide, shallow dish. Season the chicken all over with 1/2 teaspoon salt and 1/4 teaspoon pepper, dredge in breadcrumbs to coat, shake off and discard any excess crumbs. Transfer the coated breasts to a large plate.

Heat the oil in a large frying pan over medium high heat. Working in two batches, if needed, arrange chicken in the pan in a single layer and cook, flipping once, until cooked through and golden brown. This should take around 6 to 8 minutes. Transfer to plates and spoon the salsa over the top.

<u>Tip:</u>

Add chilies to the salsa for more of a kick, and a small clove of chopped garlic if you want.

Chapter 16 – Vitamin-Packed Soup

This is a brilliant, simply lunch to take to the office.

<u>You will need:</u>

1 tablespoon of extra virgin olive oil

1 medium onion, quartered and thinly sliced

3 celery stalks, thinly sliced

1 medium carrot, thinly sliced

8 medium garlic cloves, very thinly sliced

2 tablespoons of grated ginger, peeled

1 1/2 cups of mushrooms, trimmed

Salt and pepper to taste

<u>Method:</u>

Heat the oil in a large soup pot over medium heat, and stir in the onion, celery, carrot, garlic, and ginger. Gently sauté just until soft; do not allow to brown. Add a small splash of water if the pan dries out.

Stir in the pepper and 10 cups of water. Increase the heat to bring the broth to a simmer, and hold there for about 15 minutes. Add the mushrooms and salt, and gently simmer for another 5 minutes. Stir well, taste, and adjust with more salt or water if needed.

Serve with of chopped green onions, sliced watermelon radish, and/or pea shoots.

Chapter 17 – Breakfast Omelette

<u>You will need:</u>

2 whole eggs and 1 egg white

350g of beef mince

1 diced onion

Half a ripe avocado

Salt and pepper to taste

<u>Method:</u>

Sauté the beef until browned and add the onions. Remove from the pan and beat the eggs together with salt and pepper, then pour into the pan and cook until set.

Add the beef and sliced avocado and fold the omelette over. Eat immediately.

Chapter 18 – Strawberry Iced Smoothie

<u>You will need:</u>

1 scoop of protein whey powder

A handful of frozen, organic strawberries

1/2 cup of plain yogurt

1/2 cup of semi-skimmed milk (organic, rice, almond, hazelnut or coconut)

<u>Method:</u>

Add the ingredients to blender and blend until smooth. Since the fruit is frozen, there is no need to add extra ice.

Chapter 19 – BBQ Pork Chops

<u>You will need:</u>

4 pork chops, trimmed of any thick rind or fat

650ml of diet soda — cola or lemon lime flavor

2 cups of BBQ sauce

<u>Method:</u>

Combine all ingredients in a wok or deep frying pan. Cover and cook on med-high heat for 45 minutes, covered. Flip the chops every 10-15 minutes.

When all of the soda has evaporated it should form a thick sauce. Serve with green salad or a small scoop of brown rice.

Chapter 20 – Pasta Salad

<u>You will need:</u>

2 cups of cooked wholewheat pasta — omit any salt when cooking

1 cup of chopped fresh tomatoes

1 cup of peeled sliced cucumbers

1 cup of diet Italian dressing

1/2 cup of grated parmesan cheese

<u>Method:</u>

Drain and cool the pasta. Mix the rest of ingredients together with pasta and refrigerate until chilled.

You can adapt this recipe to include your favorite salad vegetables, such as radishes, raw onion, baby spinach or even a hard green apple.

Chapter 21 – Low Carb Stir Fry

<u>You will need:</u>

1 Tablespoon of sesame oil

2 boneless skinless chicken thighs

1 Tablespoon of fresh ginger, minced

1 Tablespoon of gluten-free soy sauce

A splash of water

1 teaspoon of onion powder

1/2 a teaspoon of garlic powder

1 teaspoon of red pepper flakes

1 Tablespoon of granulated sugar substitute (Splenda)

½ a small broccoli head, sliced

A handful of finely sliced savoy cabbage

A few shredded spring onion

<u>Method:</u>

Slice the chicken thighs into thin pieces or strips. In a large wok or frying pan, stir fry the chicken and minced ginger in the sesame oil for 2 - 3 minutes. Add the soy sauce, water, onion powder, garlic powder, red pepper flakes and sugar substitute. Stir well and simmer for 5 minutes.

Add the remaining vegetables and simmer for 2 minutes or until al dente. Don't allow the vegetables to become too soft.

This stir fry does not require rice or noodles — the cabbage and broccoli form the bulk of the dish.

Chapter 22 – More Smoothie Ideas

If you have a smoothie maker, this is an ideal way to make quick, nutritious meals which are packed with flavour. Choose a smoothie maker which does not filter out the fibre, as this is an important element of the meal.

Try these combinations:

Spinach and Mango:

3/4 cup plain Greek yogurt

A small bunch of spinach

1 small apple, cored and cut into chunks

Half a mango peeled and cut into chunks

A handful of ice

1 scoop protein whey powder

Banana and Cardamom:

1 cup of almond milk

1/2 tsp. ground cardamom (or crushed cardamom seeds)

1 scoop whey protein powder

1/2 a ripe banana

The juice of 1/2 lime

4 ice cubes

Cucumber and Mint:

1 scoop whey protein powder

1 cup chopped, seeded, peeled cucumber

A small bunch of chopped fresh mint

1 teaspoon of honey

6 Ice cubes

Superfood Kale:

1 scoop whey protein powder

1/2 cup chopped kale, ribs and thick stems removed

1 small stalk of celery, chopped

1/2 a ripe banana

1/4 cup apple juice

1/2 cup water

The juice of one fresh lemon

3 ice cubes

<u>Sunshine Smoothie:</u>

1 chopped, peeled mango

1 chopped, peeled nectarine

1 scoop whey protein powder

½ cup Greek yogurt

1 teaspoon grated lemon rind

½ cup water

2 Ice cubes

<u>Spinach and Citrus:</u>

1 orange peeled

1/2 ripe banana, peeled

1/2 inch thick slice pineapple with core (Skin removed)

1 handful of spinach

1 thin slice lemon (with peel)

1 scoop whey protein powder

<u>Kiwi:</u>

2 kiwis (peeled)

1 apple (peeled and cored)

2 cups fresh baby spinach

1 whole carrot (peeled)

1/2 cup water

1 scoop whey protein powder

<u>Green tea:</u>

2 medium-sized peaches

1 frozen banana

1 cup cold green tea

1 cup almond milk

1 date (optional)

A few drops vanilla extract

<u>Watermelon and ginger:</u>

1 cup watermelon, seeded and cubed

1 teaspoon fresh ginger, finely grated

1 scoop whey protein powder

1 teaspoon of fresh lime juice

<u>Strawberry and Cauliflower:</u>

1 scoop whey protein powder

1 to 2 florets cauliflower

1 cup strawberries

1 cup seedless grapes

1 cup almond milk

3 Ice cubes

<u>Strawberry and Vanilla:</u>

1 scoop whey protein powder

A handful of frozen, organic strawberries

1/2 cup plain yogurt

1/2 cup milk (semi skimmed, rice, almond, hazelnut or coconut)

<u>Smoothie Tips:</u>

- Peel, chop and freeze ripe bananas and add them directly to the smoothie maker.

- Blend fresh spinach leaves with a small amount of water and freeze them in ice cube trays to drop in with your other ingredients.

- Blend and freeze fresh herbs such as mint or coriander in the same way. Once the cubes are frozen, you can empty them into a ziplock bag and store it in the freezer to save space.

- Take advantage of seasonal berries when they are cheap. Divide them into individual portions in ziplock bags and freeze.

- Always add the ice last to prevent over-watering your smoothie.

- Avoid adding fresh citrus juice to soy-based smoothies, as it can affect the flavor.

- Freeze coconut water in ice cube trays for a flavor boost.

Conclusion

We hope you have enjoyed this guide to the Leptin diet. With a little thought and preparation, you can lose weight and feel healthier, as well as enjoying delicious, satisfying meals. There is no need to feel hungry or deprived, or to buy expensive, faddy ingredients. Many of these meals can be enjoyed by all the family, or even for dinner parties or special celebrations. Use these recipes to kick-start a new, healthier you and feel fitter, happier and have more energy!